Fast Air Fryer Recipes for Busy People

Fast and Tasty Air Fryer Recipes for your Daily Meals

By Samantha Hendrick

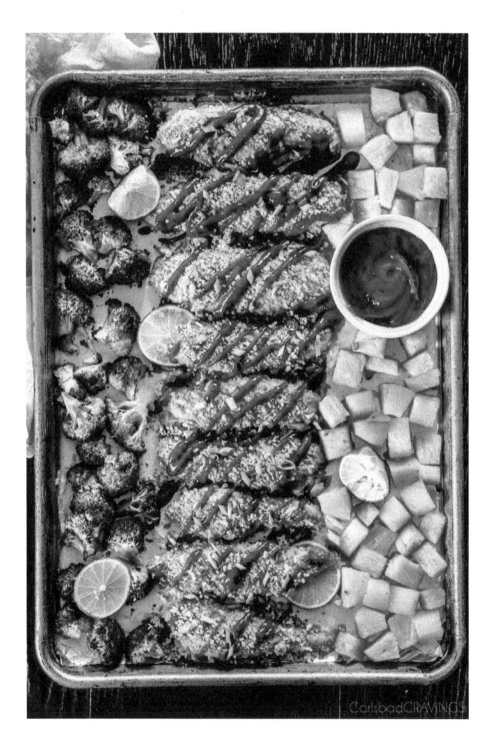

The content within this book has been derived from various sources. Please consult a licensed professional before attempting any techniques outlined in this book.

By reading this document, the reader agrees that under no circumstances is the author responsible for any losses, direct or indirect, which are incurred as a result of the use of information contained within this document, including, but not limited to, — errors, omissions, or inaccuracies.

Table of Contents

Sweet Lime 'n Chili Chicken Barbecue

Servings per Recipe: 2

Cooking Time: 40 minutes

Ingredients

- ¼ cup soy sauce /62.5ML
- 1 cup sweet chili sauce /250ML
- 1-pound chicken breasts /450G
- Juice from 2 limes, freshly squeezed

Instructions:

1) Combine all ingredients in a Ziploc bag and shake well. Allow to marinate for about 2 hours in the fridge.
2) Preheat mid-air fryer to 390° F or 199°C .
3) Place the grill pan in the air fryer.
4) Place chicken on the grill and cook for 40 to 50 minutes. Flip the chicken over every 10 minutes to cook evenly.
5) Meanwhile, Put the remaining marinade in a saucepan. Simmer before the sauce thickens.
6) Brush the cooked chicken with all the thickened marinade and serve.

Nutrition information:

- Calories per serving: 563
- Carbs: 39.2g

- Protein: 43.6g
- Fat: 25.7g

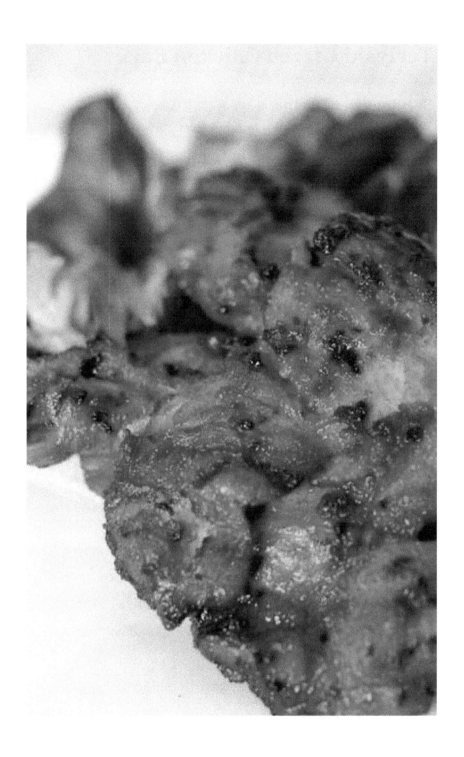

Teriyaki Glazed Chicken Bake

Servings per Recipe: 2

Cooking Time: 25 minutes

Ingredients:

- 2 tablespoons cider vinegar /30ML
- 4 skinless chicken thighs
- 1-1/2 teaspoons cornstarch /7.5G
- 1-1/2 teaspoons cold water /7.5ML
- 1/2 clove garlic, minced
- 1/4 cup white sugar /32.5G
- 1/4 cup soy sauce /62.5ML
- 1/4 teaspoon ground ginger /1.25G
- 1/8 teaspoon ground black pepper /0.625G

Instructions:

1) Grease the baking pan of the air fryer with oil using a cooking spray. Add all ingredients and mix well to coat. Spread chicken in a single layer at the bottom of the pan.
2) For 15 minutes, cook at 390° F or 199°C .
3) Turnover chicken while brushing and coating well with the sauce.
4) Cook for 15 minutes at 330° F or 166°C .
5) Serve and enjoy.

Nutrition Information:

- Calories per Serving: 267
- Carbs: 19.9g
- Protein: 24.7g
- Fat: 9.8g

Tomato, Cheese 'n Broccoli Quiche

Servings per Recipe: 2

Cooking Time: 24 minutes

Ingredients

- ½ cup Cheddar Cheese grated /65G
- ½ cup Whole Milk /125ML
- 1 Large Carrot, peeled and diced
- 1 Large Tomato, chopped
- 1 small Broccoli, cut into florets
- 1 Tsp Parsley /5G
- 1 Tsp Thyme /5G
- 2 Large Eggs
- 2 tbsp Feta Cheese /30G
- Salt & Pepper

Instructions:

1) Grease the baking pan of the air fryer with cooking spray.
2) Spread carrots, broccoli, and tomato in the baking pan.
3) For 10 minutes, cook at 330° F or 166°C .
4) Meanwhile, in a medium-sized bowl whisk eggs and milk well. Season generously with pepper and salt. Sprinkle parsley and thyme.

5) Remove the basket and add a little of the condiment. Sprinkle cheddar cheese. Pour egg mixture over vegetables and cheese.

6) Cook for another 12 minutes or until your preferred doneness.

7) Sprinkle feta cheese and allow it sit for two minutes.

8) Serve and enjoy.

Nutrition Information:

- Calories per Serving: 363
- Carbs: 23.7g
- Protein: 21.0g
- Fat: 20.4g

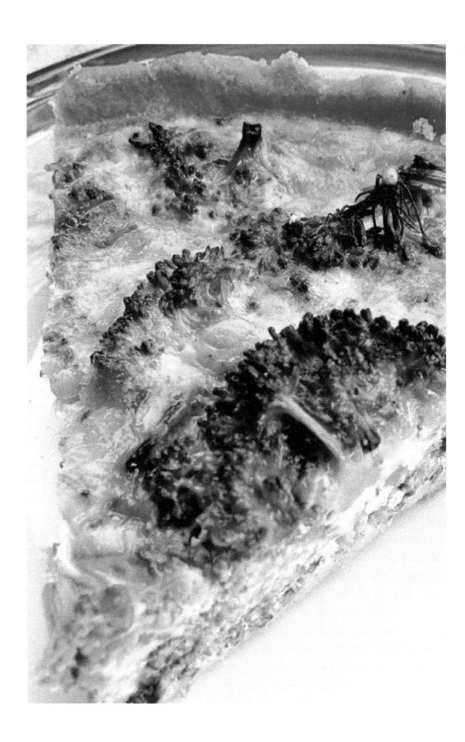

Tomato, Eggplant 'n Chicken Skewers

Servings per Recipe: 4

Cooking Time: 25 minutes

Ingredients:

- ¼ teaspoon cayenne /1.25G
- ¼ teaspoon ground cardamom /1.25G
- 1 ½ teaspoon ground turmeric /7.5G
- 1 can coconut milk /250ML
- 1 cup cherry tomatoes /130G
- 1 medium eggplant, cut into cubes
- 1 onion, cut into wedges
- 1-inch ginger, grated
- 2 pounds boneless chicken breasts, cut into cubes /900G
- 2 tablespoons fresh lime juice /30ML
- 2 tablespoons tomato paste /30ML
- 3 teaspoons lime zest /15G
- 4 cloves of garlic, minced
- Salt and pepper to taste

Instructions:

1) Place garlic, ginger, coconut milk, lime zest, lime juice, tomato paste, salt, pepper, turmeric, red pepper cayenne, cardamom, and chicken breasts in a bowl. Allow to marinate in the fridge for at least a couple of hours.

2) Preheat mid-air fryer to 390° F or 199°C .

3) Place the grill pan in a mid-air fryer.

4) Skewer the chicken cubes with eggplant, onion, and cherry tomatoes on bamboo skewers.

5) Place around the grill pan and cook for 25 minutes, turn over the chicken every 5 minutes while cooking.

Nutrition information:

- Calories per serving: 485
- Carbs:19.7 g
- Protein: 55.2g
- Fat: 20.6g

Grilled Chicken Pesto

Servings per Recipe: 8

Cooking Time: 30 Minutes

Ingredients:

- 1 ¾ cup commercial pesto /208G
- 8 chicken thighs
- Salt and pepper to taste

Instructions:

1) Place all Ingredients within the Ziploc bag and allow to marinate in the fridge for some hours.
2) Preheat mid-air fryer to 390° F or 199°C .
3) Place the grill pan accessory inside the air fryer.
4) Grill the chicken for about half an hour.
5) Flip the chicken every 10 minutes for even grilling.

Nutrition information:

- Calories per serving: 477
- Carbs: 3.8g
- Protein: 32.6g
- Fat: 36.8g

Grilled Chicken Recipe From Jamaica

Servings per Recipe: 2

Cooking Time: 30 Minutes

Ingredients:

- ¼ cup pineapple chunks /32.5G
- 1 tablespoon vegetable oil /15ML
- 2 whole chicken thighs
- 3 teaspoons lime juice /15ML
- 4 tablespoons jerk seasoning /60G

Instructions:

1) Mix well all ingredients in a bowl. Marinate inside the refrigerator for 3 hours.
2) Thread chicken pieces and pineapples alternatively in skewers. Place on skewer rack in the air fryer.
3) For half an hour, cook at 360° F or 183°C . turn skewer after half the cooking time has passed.
4) Serve and enjoy.

Nutrition Information:

- Calories per Serving: 579
- Carbs: 36.3g
- Protein: 25.7g
- Fat: 36.7g

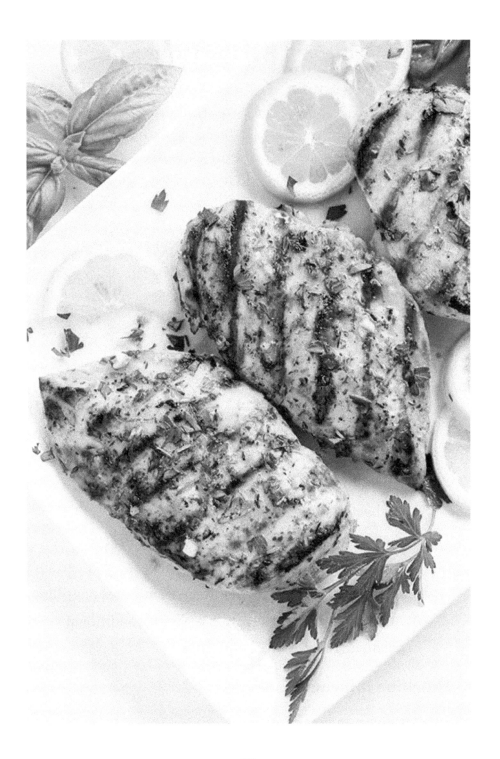

Grilled Chicken Recipe from Korea

Servings per Recipe: 4

Cooking Time: 30 Minutes

Ingredients:

- ½ cup gochujang /65G
- ½ teaspoon fresh ground black pepper /2.5G
- 1 scallion, sliced thinly
- 1 teaspoon salt /5G
- 2 pounds chicken wings /900G

Instructions:

1) Put the chicken wings in a Ziploc bag, add salt, pepper, and gochujang sauce. Mix to combine all ingredients.
2) Allow to marinate within the fridge for at least a couple of hours.
3) Preheat mid-air fryer to 390° F or 199°C .
4) Place the grill pan accessory inside the air fryer.
5) Grill the chicken wings for 30 minutes making certain to turn over the chicken after every 10 minutes of grilling.
6) Add scallions to the top and serve with additional gochujang.

Nutrition information:

- Calories per serving: 278

- Carbs: 0.8g
- Protein: 50.1g
- Fat: 8.2g

Grilled Chicken Recipe from Morocco

Servings per Recipe: 4

Cooking Time: 20 Minutes

Ingredients:

- 1-pound skinless, boneless chicken thighs, cut into 2" pieces /450G
- 2 garlic cloves, chopped
- 2 teaspoons ground cumin /10G
- 2 teaspoons paprika /10G
- 3 tablespoons plain yogurt /45ML
- 4 garlic cloves, finely chopped
- Kosher salt
- Kosher salt
- Vegetable oil (for grilling)
- Warm pita bread, labneh (Lebanese strained yogurt), chopped tomatoes, and fresh mint leaves (for serving)
- 1/2 cup finely chopped fresh flat-leaf parsley /65G
- 1/3 cup organic olive oil /83ML
- 1/4 teaspoon crushed red pepper flakes /32.5G

Instructions:

1) Blend the garlic, salt, and oil until creamy. Add yogurt and continue blending until emulsified. Transfer to a bowl set aside inside a fridge.

2) Soak chicken in red pepper flakes, paprika, cumin, parsley, and garlic. Marinate for several hours in the refrigerator.

3) Thread chicken in skewers and set in the skewer rack of the air fryer.

4) Cook at 390° F or 199°C for 10 minutes. Turnover skewers after 5 minutes of cooking.

5) Use dip for side, serve and enjoy.

Nutrition Information:

- Calories per Serving: 343
- Carbs: 8.1g
- Protein: 28.0g
- Fat: 22.0g

Grilled Chicken Wings with Curry-Yogurt Sauce

Servings per Recipe: 4

Cooking Time: 35 minutes

Ingredients:

- ½ cup plain yogurt /125ML
- 1 tablespoon curry powder /15G
- 2 pounds chicken wings /900G
- Salt and pepper to taste

Instructions:

1) Season the chicken wings with yogurt, curry powder, salt and pepper. Mix properly to combine everything.
2) Allow to marinate in the fridge for about 120 minutes.
3) Preheat the air fryer to 390° F or 199°C .
4) Place the grill pan accessory in the air fryer.
5) Grill the chicken for 35 minutes and flip the chicken halfway through cooking time.

Nutrition information:

- Calories per serving: 301
- Carbs: 3.3g
- Protein: 51.3g
- Fat: 9.2g

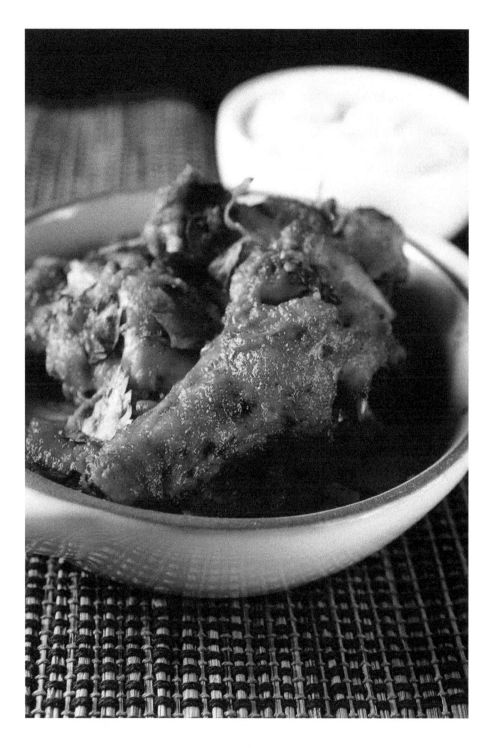

Chicken in Packets Southwest Style

Servings per Recipe: 4

Cooking Time: 40 minutes

Ingredients:

- 1 can black beans, rinsed and drained
- 1 cup cilantro, chopped /130G
- 1 cup commercial salsa /130G
- 1 cup corn kernels, frozen /130G
- 1 cup Mexican cheese blend, shredded /130G
- 4 chicken breasts
- 4 lime wedges
- 4 teaspoons taco seasoning /20G
- Salt and pepper to taste

Instructions:

1) Preheat air fryer to 390° F or 199°C .
2) Place the grill pan accessory in the air fryer.
3) Place the chicken breasts on a large aluminium foil, and season with salt and pepper to taste.
4) Add the corn, commercial salsa beans, and taco seasoning.
5) Wrap the foil and crumple the sides.
6) Place on the grill pan and cook for 40 minutes.
7) Before serving, top with cheese, cilantro and lime wedges.

Nutrition information:

- Calories per serving: 837
- Carbs: 47.5g
- Protein: 80.1g
- Fat: 36.2g

Chicken Kebab with Aleppo 'n Yogurt

Servings per Recipe: 2

Cooking Time: 20 minutes

Ingredients:

- 1 tablespoon Aleppo pepper /15G

- 1 tablespoon extra-virgin olive oil /15ML

- 1 tablespoon red wine vinegar /15ML

- 1 tablespoon tomato paste /15ML

- 1 teaspoon coarse kosher salt /5G

- 1 teaspoon freshly ground black pepper /5G

- 3 garlic cloves, peeled, flattened

- 1-pound skinless boneless chicken (thighs and/or breast halves), cut into 1 1/4-inch cube /450G

- 1 unpeeled lemon; 1/2 thinly sliced into rounds, 1/2 cut into wedges for serving

- 1/3 cup plain whole-milk Greek-style yogurt /88ML

Instructions:

1) Add all ingredients to a bowl and mix properly. Place in a fridge and allow to marinate for nothing short of an hour.
2) Skewer chicken and place in the air fryer skewer rack.
3) For 10 minutes, cook at 360° F or 183°C . Turnover skewers after 5 minutes of cooking.
4) Serve with lemon wedges and enjoy.

Nutrition Information:

- Calories per Serving: 336
- Carbs: 7.0g
- Protein: 53.6g
- Fat: 10.4g

Chicken Meatballs with Miso-Ginger

Servings per Recipe: 4

Cooking Time: 10 Minutes

Ingredients:

- 1 1/2 teaspoons white miso paste /7.5ML
- 1 large egg
- 1 teaspoon finely grated ginger /5G
- 1/4 cup panko (Japanese breadcrumbs), or fresh breadcrumbs /32.5 g
- 1/4 teaspoon kosher salt /1.25G
- 2 tablespoons sliced scallions /30G
- 2 teaspoons low-sodium soy sauce /10ML
- 3/4-pound ground chicken /338G

Instructions:

1) Add soy sauce, miso paste, and ginger to a medium-sized bowl. Mix all ingredients. Set aside.
2) Add ground chicken, large egg, scallions, and salt to another bowl and mix well with hands. Add panko and half of the sauce. Mix well continuously.
3) Evenly form 12 balls with the mix. Thread into 4 skewers.
4) Place on skewer rack.

5) Cook for 2 minutes at 390° F or 199°C . Baste with remaining sauce, turnover and cook for another 2 minutes. Baste with sauce again and cook for another 2 minutes.

6) Serve and enjoy.

Nutrition Information:

- Calories per Serving: 145
- Carbs: 4.2g
- Protein: 17.4g
- Fat: 8.2g

Chicken Pot Pie with Coconut Milk

Serves: 8

Cooking Time: 30 Minutes

Ingredients:

- ¼ small onion, chopped
- ½ cup broccoli, chopped/65G
- ¾ cup coconut milk /188ML
- 1 cup chicken broth /250ML
- 1/3 cup coconut flour /43G
- 1-pound ground chicken /450G
- 2 cloves of garlic, minced
- 2 tablespoons butter /30G
- 4 ½ tablespoons butter, melted 75ML
- 4 eggs
- Salt and pepper to taste

Instructions:

1) Preheat the air fryer for 5 minutes.
2) Place 2 tablespoons of butter, broccoli, onion, garlic, coconut milk, chicken broth, and ground chicken inside a baking dish. Mix well. Season with salt and pepper to taste.
3) Add the butter, coconut flour, and eggs into a mixing bowl. Mix well.

4) Sprinkle the top of the chicken and broccoli mixture with the coconut flour dough.

5) Place the dish inside the air fryer.

6) Cook for 30 minutes at 325° F or 163°C .

Nutrition information:

- Calories per serving: 366
- Carbohydrates: 3.4g
- Protein: 21.8g
- Fat: 29.5g

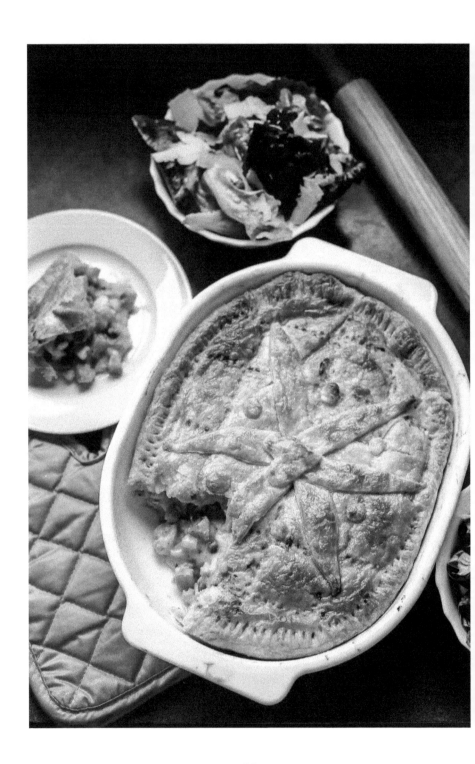

Chicken Roast with Pineapple Salsa

Servings per Recipe: 2

Cooking Time: 45 minutes

Ingredients:

- ¼ cup extra virgin organic olive oil /62.5ML
- ¼ cup freshly chopped cilantro /32.5G
- 1 avocado, diced
- 1-pound boneless chicken breasts /450G
- 2 cups canned pineapples /260G
- 2 teaspoons honey /10ML
- Juice from 1 lime
- Salt and pepper to taste

Instructions:

1) Preheat the air fryer to 390° F or 199°C .
2) Place the grill pan accessory in the air fryer.
3) Place chicken breast in a bowl. Season with lime juice, organic olive oil, honey, salt, and pepper.
4) Place on the grill pan and cook for 45 minutes.
5) Flip the chicken every 10 minutes for even grilling.
6) Once the chicken is cooked, serve with pineapples, cilantro, and avocado.

Nutrition information:

- Calories per serving: 744
- Carbs: 57.4g
- Protein: 54.7g
- Fat: 32.8g

Spinach-Egg with Coconut Milk Casserole

Serves: 6

Cooking Time: 20 minutes

Ingredients:

- ¼ cup coconut milk /62.5ML
- 1 onion, chopped
- 1 teaspoon garlic powder /5G
- 12 large eggs, beaten
- 2 tablespoons coconut oil /30ML
- 3 cups spinach, chopped /390G
- Salt and pepper to taste

Instructions:

1) Preheat the air fryer for 5 minutes.
2) Combine all ingredients except the spinach in a mixing bowl. Whisk until well combined.
3) Place the spinach in a baking dish and pour the egg mixture
4) Place in mid-air fryer chamber and cook for 20 minutes at 310° F or 155°C .

Nutrition information:

- Calories per serving:185

- Carbohydrates: 3.2g
- Protein: 6.9g
- Fat: 16.1g

Sriracha-Ginger Chicken

Servings per Recipe: 3

Cooking Time: 25 minutes

Ingredients:

- ¼ cup fish sauce /62.5ML
- ¼ cup sriracha /62.5ML
- ½ cup light brown sugar /65G
- ½ cup rice vinegar /125ML
- 1 ½ pounds chicken breasts, pounded /675G
- 1/3 cup hot chili paste /83ML
- 2 teaspoons grated and peeled ginger /10G

Instructions:

1) Place all ingredients inside a Ziploc bag. Place in a fridge for some hours.
2) Preheat air fryer to 390° F or 199°C .
3) Place the grill pan in the air fryer.
4) Grill the chicken for 25 minutes.
5) Flip the chicken over every 10 minutes for even grilling.
6) Meanwhile, pour the marinade inside a saucepan and warmth over a medium flame before the sauce thickens.
7) Before serving the chicken, brush using the sriracha sauce.

Nutrition information:

- Calories per serving: 415
- Carbs: 5.4g
- Protein: 49.3g
- Fat: 21.8g

Sriracha-vinegar Marinated Chicken

Servings per Recipe: 4

Cooking Time: 40 minutes

Ingredients:

- ¼ cup Thai fish sauce /62.5ML
- ¼ cups sriracha sauce 62.5ML
- ½ cup rice vinegar /125ML
- 1 tablespoons sugar /15G
- 2 garlic cloves, minced
- 2 pounds chicken breasts
- Juice from 1 lime, freshly squeezed
- Salt and pepper to taste

Instructions:

1) Place all ingredients in a Ziploc bag except for the corn. Allow to marinate in the fridge for at least 2 hours.
2) Preheat the air fryer to 390° F or 199°C .
3) Place the grill pan in the air fryer.
4) Grill the chicken for 40 minutes, turn over the chicken to grill evenly.
5) Meanwhile, pour the marinade in a saucepan and place the saucepan over medium flame until it thickens.
6) Brush the chicken with the sauce. Serve with cucumbers if desired.

Nutrition information:

- Calories per serving: 427
- Carbs: 6.7g
- Protein: 49.1g
- Fat: 22.6g

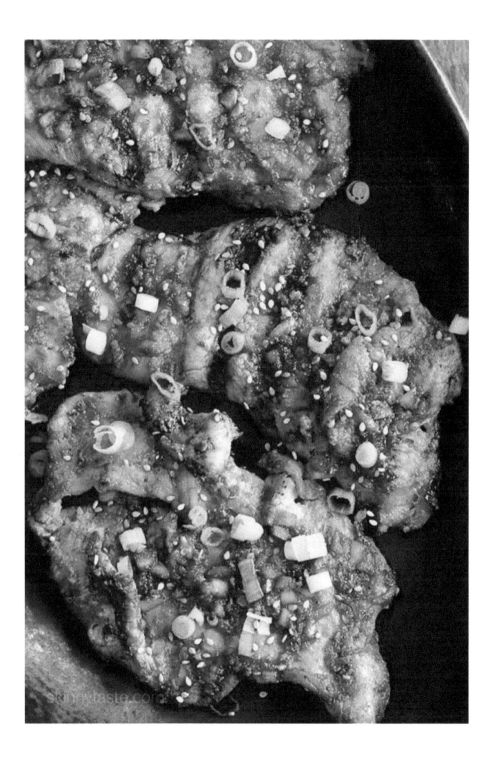

Sticky-Sweet Chicken BBQ

Servings per Recipe: 2

Cooking Time: 40 minutes

Ingredients:

- ½ cup balsamic vinegar /125ML
- ½ cup soy sauce /125ML
- 1-pound chicken drumsticks /450G
- 2 cloves of garlic, minced
- 2 green onion, sliced thinly
- 2 tablespoons sesame seeds /30G
- 3 tablespoons honey /45ML

Instructions:

1) Place the soy sauce, balsamic vinegar, honey, garlic, and chicken in a Ziploc bag, mix to combine. Place in the fridge for 30 minutes and allow to marinate.
2) Preheat air fryer to 330° F or 166°C .
3) Place the grill pan in the air fryer.
4) Place on the grill and cook for 30-40 minutes. Turnover the chicken every 10 minutes to grill evenly.
5) Meanwhile, Place the marinade in a saucepan. Simmer before the sauce thickens.

6) Once the chicken is cooked, brush with all the thickened marinade and garnish with sesame seeds and green onions.

Nutrition information:

- Calories per serving: 594
- Carbs: 43.7g
- Protein: 48.7g
- Fat: 24.9g

Cheesy BBQ Tater Tot

Servings per Recipe: 6

Cooking Time: 20 minutes

Ingredients:

- ½ cup shredded Cheddar /65G
- 12 slices of bacon
- 1-lb frozen tater tots, defrosted /450G
- 2 tbsp. chives /30G
- Ranch dressing, for serving

Instructions:

1) Thread one end of the strip of bacon on a steel skewer, thread a tater tot, and then flip the bacon over the tater tot, pushing it down the skewer. Repeat until you have a twirling bacon-and-tot.
2) Place skewer in your air fryer and cook for 10 minutes at 360° F or 183°C . Turn over skewer regularly while cooking.
3) Serve skewers on a plate, sprinkle cheese and chives on it.
4) Use ranch dressing for the side.

Nutrition Information:

- Calories per Serving: 337
- Carbs: 17.2g

- Protein: 11.5g
- Fat: 29.1g

Chives 'n Thyme Spiced Veggie Burger

Serves: 8

Cooking Time: 15

Ingredients:

- ¼ cup desiccated coconut /32.5G
- ½ cup oats /65G
- ½ pound cauliflower, steamed and diced /225G
- 1 cup bread crumbs /130G
- 1 flax egg (1 flaxseed egg + 3 tablespoon or 45ML water)
- 1 teaspoon mustard powder /5G
- 2 teaspoons chives /10G
- 2 teaspoons coconut oil melted /10ML
- 2 teaspoons garlic, minced /10G
- 2 teaspoons parsley /10G
- 2 teaspoons thyme /10G
- 3 tablespoons plain flour/45G
- salt and pepper to taste

Instructions:

1) Preheat air fryer to 390° F or 199°C .
2) Place cauliflower in a large tea towel and squeeze out surplus water. Remove cauliflower from the tea towel and place in a bowl, add ingredients except for bread crumbs. Mix well.

3) Using your hands make 8 burger patties.
4) Turn the patties in bread crumbs, place them in the air fryer basket and avoid overlapping.
5) Cook until patties are crisp.

Nutrition information:

- Calories per serving: 70
- Carbohydrates: 10.85g
- Protein: 2.51g
- Fat: 1.85g

Coconut Battered Cauliflower Bites

Serves: 4

Cooking Time: 20 Minutes

Ingredients:

- salt and pepper to taste
- 1 flax egg (1 tablespoon flaxseed meal or 15G + 3 tablespoon or 45ML water)
- 1 small cauliflower, cut into florets
- 1 teaspoon mixed spice /5G
- ½ teaspoon mustard powder /2.5G
- 2 tablespoons maple syrup /30ML
- 1 clove of garlic, minced
- 2 tablespoons soy sauce /30ML
- 1/3 cup oats flour /43G
- 1/3 cup plain flour /43G
- 1/3 cup desiccated coconut /43G

Instructions

1) Preheat mid-air fryer to 400° F or 205°C .
2) Add oats, flour, and desiccated coconut in a bowl and mix well. Season with salt and pepper and allow to set.
3) Place flax egg in a bowl, add a pinch of salt and set aside.
4) Place cauliflower (florets) in a bowl, add mixed spice and mustard powder. Mix well.

5) Drench the florets inside the flax egg and then turn them over in the flour mixture.

6) Place inside air fryer basket and cook for 15 minutes.

7) Place a large saucepan over medium heat, add maple syrup, garlic, and soy sauce. Allow to boil until the sauce thickens.

8) Remove the florets from the air fryer pour them inside the saucepan. Turn the florets to coat, place in mid-air fryer and cook again for 5 more minutes.

Nutrition information:

- Calories per serving: 154
- Carbohydrates: 27.88g
- Protein: 4.69g
- Fat:2.68 g

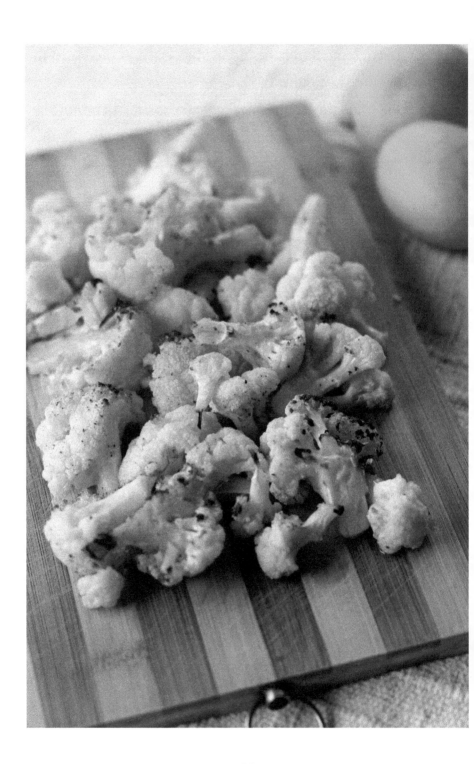

Creamy 'n Cheese Broccoli Bake

Servings per Recipe: 2

Cooking Time: 30 Minutes

Ingredients:

- 1-pound fresh broccoli, coarsely chopped /450G
- 2 tablespoons all-purpose flour /43G
- salt to taste
- 1 tablespoon dry bread crumbs /15G
- 1/2 large onion, coarsely chopped
- 1/2 (14 ounces or 120G) can evaporated milk, divided
- 1/2 cup cubed sharp Cheddar cheese /65G
- 1-1/2 teaspoons butter /7.5G
- 1/4 cup water /62.5ML

Instructions:

1) Oil baking pan lightly with cooking spray. Add milk and flour to the pan and cook for 5 minutes at 360° F or 183°C . After cooking add broccoli and the remaining milk. Mix well and cook for another 5 minutes.
2) Add in cheese and mix well until melted.
3) Add butter and bread crumbs to a small bowl. Sprinkle these on top of broccoli.
4) Cook for 20 Minutes at 360° F or 183°C or until tops are lightly browned.

5) Dish out and enjoy.

Nutrition Information:

- Calories per Serving: 444
- Carbs: 37.3g
- Protein: 23.1g
- Fat: 22.4g

Creole Seasoned Vegetables

Servings per Recipe: 5

Cooking Time: 15 minutes

Ingredients:

- ¼ cup honey /62.5ML

- ¼ cup yellow mustard /32.5G

- 1 large red bell pepper, sliced

- 1 teaspoon black pepper /5G

- 1 teaspoon salt /5G

- 2 large yellow squash, cut into ½ inch thick slices

- 2 medium zucchinis, cut into ½ inch thick slices

- 2 teaspoons creole seasoning /10G

- 2 teaspoons smoked paprika /10G

- 3 tablespoons olive oil /45ML

Instructions:

1) Preheat mid-air fryer to 330° F or 166°C .
2) Set the grill pan in the mid-air fryer.
3) Grab a Ziploc bag, add zucchini, squash, red bell pepper, extra virgin olive oil, salt and pepper. Shake the bag vigorously so that all vegetables are seasoned.
4) Place on the grill pan and cook for 15 minutes.

5) For the sauce, add mustard, honey, paprika, and creole seasoning. Mix well. Season with salt to taste.

6) Dish out the vegetables and dress using the sauce.

Nutrition information:

- Calories per serving: 164
- Carbs: 21.5g
- Protein: 2.6g
- Fat: 8.9g

Baked Scallops with Garlic Aioli

Servings per Recipe: 4

Cooking Time: 10

Ingredients:

- 1 cup bread crumbs /130g
- 1/4 cup chopped parsley /32.5g
- 16 sea scallops, rinsed and drained
- 2 shallots, chopped
- 3 pinches ground nutmeg
- 4 tablespoons essential olive oil /60ml
- 5 cloves garlic, minced
- 5 tablespoons butter, melted /75ml
- Salt and pepper to taste

Instructions:

1) Lightly grease your baking pan with oil.
2) In a bowl, mix shallots, garlic, melted butter, and scallops. Season with pepper, salt, and nutmeg.
3) In another bowl, properly whisk organic olive oil and bread crumbs. Sprinkle over scallops.
4) Cook on 3900 F or 199°C for 10 minutes until lightly brown.
5) Dress with a sprinkle of parsley and serve.

Nutrition Information:

- Calories per Serving: 452
- Carbs: 29.8g
- Protein: 15.2g
- Fat: 30.2g

Basil 'n Lime-Chili Clams

Servings per Recipe: 3

Cooking Time: 15 minutes

Ingredients:

- ½ cup basil leaves /65g
- ½ cup tomatoes, chopped /65g
- 1 tablespoon fresh lime juice /15ml
- 25 littleneck clams
- 4 cloves of garlic, minced
- 6 tablespoons unsalted butter /90g
- Salt and pepper to taste

Instructions:

1) Prewarm the air fryer to 3900 F or 199°C.
2) Place a fitting grill pan in the air fryer.
3) Place all ingredients in a large foil and fold over. Tuck the edges.
4) Place in a grill pan and cook for 15 minutes.
5) Serve with bread.

Nutrition information:

- Calories per serving: 163
- Carbs: 4.1g
- Protein: 1.7g

- Fat: 15.5g

Bass Filet in Coconut Sauce

Serves: 4

Cooking Time: 15

Ingredients:

- ¼ cup coconut milk
- ½ pound bass fillet
- 1 tablespoon organic olive oil /15ml
- 2 tablespoons jalapeno, chopped /30g
- 2 tablespoons lime juice, freshly squeezed /30ml
- 3 tablespoons parsley, chopped /45g
- Salt and pepper to taste

Instructions:

1) Warm mid-air fryer for 5 minutes.
2) Spice the bass with salt and pepper to taste.
3) Brush the top with organic olive oil.
4) Place in the air fryer and cook for 15 at 3500 F or 177°C.
5) Meanwhile, in a saucepan, add coconut milk, lime juice, jalapeno and parsley.
6) Cook over medium heat.
7) Serve the fish with coconut sauce.

Nutrition information:

- Calories per serving: 139
- Carbohydrates: 2.7g
- Protein: 8.7g
- Fat: 10.3

Beer Battered Cod Filet

Servings per Recipe: 2

Cooking Time: 15 minutes

Ingredients:

- ½ cup all-purpose flour /65g
- ¾ teaspoon baking powder /3.75g
- 1 ¼ cup lager beer /312.5ml
- 2 cod fillets
- 2 eggs, beaten
- Salt and pepper to taste

Instructions:

1) Preheat mid-air fryer to 3900 F or 199°C .
2) Pat the fish fillets dry with a paper towel and set them aside.
3) Combine all other ingredients in a bowl to form a batter.
4) Dip the fillets in the batter and place them in the double layer rack.
5) Cook for 15 minutes.

Nutrition information:

- Calories per serving: 229
- Carbs: 33.2g
- Protein: 31.1g

- Fat: 10.2g

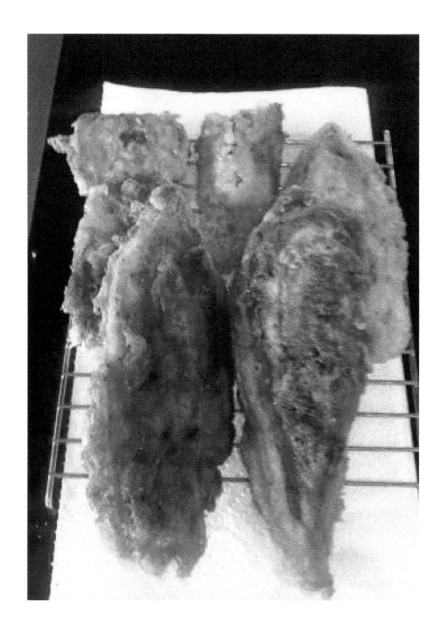

Lemony-Sage on Grilled Swordfish

Servings per Recipe: 2

Cooking Time: 16 minutes

Ingredients:

- ½ lemon, sliced thinly in rounds
- 1 tbsp fresh lemon juice /15ML
- 1 tsp parsley /5G
- 1 zucchini, peeled after which thinly sliced in lengths
- 1/2-pound swordfish, sliced into 2-inch chunks /225G
- 2 tbsp extra virgin olive oil /30ML
- 6-8 sage leaves
- salt and pepper to taste

Instructions:

1) Mix freshly squeezed lemon juice, parsley, and sliced swordfish in a shallow bowl. Stir well to coat and season with pepper and salt as you prefer. Marinate for about 10 minutes.

2) Place a zucchini over a flat surface. Add one part of fish and sage leaf in the middle, roll up zucchini and then thread on a skewer. Repeat the process until all ingredients have been exhausted.

3) Brush with oil and place on a skewer rack in the air fryer.

4) For 8 minutes, cook at 390° F or 199°C . Cook in batches preferably.

5) Serve and enjoy with fresh lemon slices.

Nutrition Information:

- Calories per Serving: 297
- Carbs: 3.7g
- Protein: 22.8g
- Fat: 21.2g

Lime 'n Chat masala Rubbed Snapper

Servings per Recipe: 2

Cooking Time: 25 minutes

Ingredients:

- 1/3 cup chat masala /43G
- 1-1/2 pounds whole fish, cut by 50 per cent /675G
- 2 tablespoons organic olive oil /30ML
- 3 tablespoons fresh lime juice /45ML
- Salt to taste

Instructions:

1) Preheat mid-air fryer to 390° F or 199°C .
2) Place the grill pan in the air fryer.
3) Place fish on a flat surface and season the fish with salt, chat masala and lime juice.
4) Brush with oil
5) Place the fish in the air fryer's basket lined with foil.
6) Cook for 25 minutes. Turn over halfway through cooking time.

Nutrition information:

- Calories per serving:308
- Carbs: 0.7g
- Protein: 35.2g

- Fat: 17.4g

Lime, Oil 'n Leeks on Grilled Swordfish

Servings per Recipe: 4

Cooking Time: 20 Minutes

Ingredients:

- 2 tablespoons olive oil /30ML
- 3 tablespoons lime juice /45ML
- 4 medium leeks, cut into an inch long
- 4 swordfish steaks
- Salt and pepper to taste

Instructions:

1) Preheat air fryer to 390° F or 199°C .
2) Place the grill pan in the air fryer.
3) Season the swordfish with salt, pepper and lime juice.
4) Brush the fish with extra virgin olive oil
5) Place fish fillets in a grill pan and garnish with leeks.
6) Grill for 20 minutes.

Nutrition information:

- Calories per serving: 611
- Carbs: 14.6g
- Protein: 48g
- Fat: 40g

Lobster-Spinach Lasagna Recipe from Maine

Servings per Recipe: 6

Cooking Time: 50 minutes

Ingredients:

- 1 (16 ounces or 480G) jar Alfredo pasta sauce
- 1 cup shredded Cheddar cheese /130G
- 1 egg
- 1 pound cooked and cubed lobster meat /450G
- 1 tablespoon chopped fresh parsley /15G
- 1/2 (15 ounces or 450G) container ricotta cheese
- 1/2 cup grated Parmesan cheese /65G
- 1/2 cup shredded mozzarella cheese /65G
- 1/2 medium onion, minced
- 1/2 teaspoon freshly ground black pepper /2.5G
- 1-1/2 teaspoons minced garlic /7.5G
- 5-ounce package baby spinach leaves /150G
- 8 no-boil lasagna noodles

Instructions:

1) Mix 50% of Parmesan, half mozzarella, 50% of cheddar, egg, and ricotta cheese in a medium-sized bowl. Sprinkle pepper, parsley, garlic, and onion.

2) Lightly grease baking pan of air fryer with cooking spray using any oil of your choice.

3) Spread ½ of the Alfredo sauce in the baking pan. Sprinkle a single layer of lasagna noodles on it, also place 1/3 of lobster meat, 1/3 of ricotta cheese mixture, 1/3 of spinach. Repeat the layering process until all ingredients are exhausted.

4) Sprinkle remaining cheese on top. Shake pan for ingredients to set and for air bubbles to burst. Cover pan with foil.

5) Cook at 360° F for 30 minutes or 183°C .

6) Remove foil and cook for an additional 10 minutes at the same temperature until tops are lightly brown and the middle is set.

7) Let it cool for 10 minutes.

8) Serve, eat and enjoy.

Nutrition Information:

- Calories per Serving: 558
- Carbs: 20.4g
- Protein: 36.8g
- Fat: 36.5g

Mango Salsa on Fish Tacos

Servings per Recipe: 4

Cooking Time: 10

Ingredients:

- ½ cup mango salsa of your choice /65G
- 1 cup corn kernels /130G
- 1 cup mixed greens /130G
- 1 red bell pepper, seeded and diced
- 1 yellow onion, peeled and diced
- 4 large burrito-size tortillas
- 4 pieces of fish fillets
- Juice from ½ lemon
- Salt and pepper to taste

Instructions:

1) Preheat the air fryer to 330° F or 166°C .
2) Season the fish with freshly squeezed lemon juice, salt and pepper to taste.
3) Place seasoned fish on the double layer rack.
4) Cook for 10 minutes.
5) Place tortillas over a flat surface, add fish fillet, onions, pepper, corn kernels, and mixed greens. This will make 4 tortilla wraps
6) Serve with mango salsa.

Nutrition information:

- Calories per serving: 378
- Carbs: 36g
- Protein: 26.8g
- Fat: 14g

Pepper-Pineapple with Butter-Sugar Glaze

Servings per Recipe: 2

Cooking Time: 10 Minutes

Ingredients:

- 1 medium-sized pineapple, peeled and sliced
- 1 red bell pepper, seeded and julienned
- 1 teaspoon brown sugar /5G
- 2 teaspoons melted butter /10ML
- Salt to taste

Instructions

1) Preheat mid-air fryer to 390° F or 199°C .
2) Place the grill pan in the air fryer.
3) Mix all ingredients in the Ziploc bag and shake.
4) Place on the grill pan and cook for 10 minutes, flip the pineapples every 5 minutes.

Nutrition information:

- Calories per serving: 295
- Carbs: 57g
- Protein: 1g
- Fat: 8g

Pita 'n Tomato Pesto Casserole

Servings per Recipe: 3

Cooking Time: 5 minutes

Ingredients:

- 1 Roma (plum) tomatoes, chopped
- 1 tablespoon and 1-1/2 teaspoons extra virgin olive oil /22.5ML
- 1 tablespoon grated Parmesan cheese /15G
- 1/2 bunch spinach, rinsed and chopped
- 1/4 cup crumbled feta cheese /32.5G
- 2 fresh mushrooms, sliced
- 3 (6 inches) whole-wheat pita bread
- 3-ounce sun-dried tomato pesto /90G
- ground black pepper to taste

Instructions:

1) Grease baking pan of air fryer with cooking spray.
2) Evenly spread tomato pesto on pita bread. Place one pita bread on the bottom of the pan, add 1/3 of Parmesan, feta, mushrooms, spinach, and tomatoes. Season with pepper and drizzle with extra virgin olive oil.
3) Cook for 5 minutes at 390° F or 199°C until tops crisped.
4) Repeat the process for the remaining pita bread.
5) Serve and luxuriate in.

Nutrition Information:

- Calories per Serving: 367
- Carbs: 41.6g

Protein: 11.6g

- Fat: 17.1g

Pull-Apart Bread With Garlicky Oil

Serves: 2

Cooking Time: 10 Minutes

Ingredients:

- 1 large vegan bread loaf
- 2 tablespoons garlic puree /30ML
- 2 tablespoons nutritional yeast /30G
- 2 tablespoons olive oil /30ML
- 2 teaspoons chives /10G
- salt and pepper to taste

Instructions:

1) Preheat air fryer to 357° F or 181°C .
2) Slice the bread loaf making sure that you don't slice over the bread.
3) Add the extra virgin olive oil, garlic puree, and nutritional yeast.
4) Pour over the mixture, now place the bread.
5) Sprinkle with chopped chives and season with salt and pepper.
6) Place inside mid-air fryer and cook for 10 or before the garlic is thoroughly cooked.

Nutrition information:

- Calories per serving: 219
- Carbohydrates: 16.07g
- Protein: 6.65g
- Fat: 14.26g

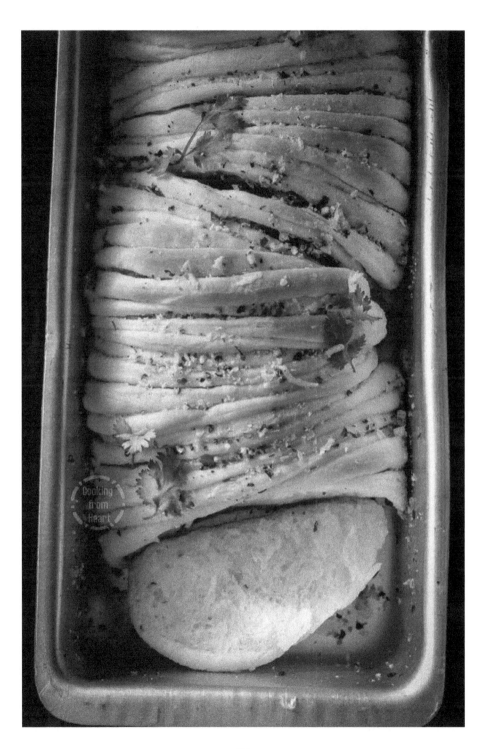

Quinoa Bowl with Lime-Sriracha

Servings per Recipe: 4

Cooking Time: 10 Minutes

Ingredients:

- ¼ cup soy sauce /62.5ML
- 1 block extra firm tofu
- 1 red bell pepper, sliced
- 1 tablespoon sriracha /15ML
- 1-pound fresh broccoli florets, blanched /450G
- 2 cups quinoa, cooked according to package instruction /260G
- 2 tablespoons lime juice /30ML
- 2 tablespoons sesame oil /30ML
- 3 medium carrots, peeled and thinly sliced
- 3 tablespoons molasses /45G
- 8 ounces spinach, blanched /240G
- Salt and pepper to taste

Instructions:

1) Season tofu with sesame oil, salt and pepper.
2) Place the grill pan accessory in the mid-air fryer.
3) Place the seasoned tofu about the grill pan accessory.
4) Close the air fryer and cook for 10 minutes at 330°F or 166°C .

5) Stir the tofu to brown all sides evenly.

6) Set aside and arrange the Buddha bowl.

7) In a mixing bowl, combine the soy sauce, molasses, lime juice and sriracha. Set aside.

8) Place quinoa in bowls and top with broccoli, carrots, red bell pepper, and spinach.

9) Top in tofu and drizzle while using sauce last.

Nutrition information:

- Calories per serving: 157
- Carbs: 17g
- Protein: 9g
- Fat: 6g

Roasted Bell Peppers 'n Onions in a Salad

Serves: 4

Cooking Time: 10

Ingredients:

- ½ lemon, juiced
- 1 tablespoon baby capers /15G
- 1 tablespoon extra-virgin essential olive oil /15ML
- 1 teaspoon paprika /5G
- 2 large red onions sliced
- 2 yellow pepper, sliced
- 4 long red pepper, sliced
- 6 cloves of garlic, crushed
- 6 plum tomatoes, halved
- salt and pepper to taste

Instructions:

1) Preheat the air fryer to 420° F or 216°C .
2) Place the tomatoes, onions, peppers, and garlic in a mixing bowl.
3) Add in the extra virgin organic olive oil, paprika, and freshly squeezed lemon juice. Season with salt and pepper to taste.

4) Transfer into the air fryer lined with aluminium foil and cook for 10 minutes or before the edges from the vegetables have brown.

5) Place inside a salad bowl and add the baby capers. Mix well to combine all ingredients.

Nutrition information:

- Calories per serving: 163
- Carbohydrates: 36.56g
- Protein: 3.58g
- Fat:2.08 g

Grilled Spicy Carne Asada

Servings per Recipe: 2

Cooking Time: 50 minutes

Ingredients:

- 1 chipotle pepper, chopped
- 1 dried ancho chilies, chopped
- 1 tablespoon coriander seeds /15G
- 1 tablespoon cumin /15G
- 1 tablespoon soy sauce /15ML
- 2 slices skirt steak
- 2 tablespoons Asian fish sauce /30ML
- 2 tablespoons brown sugar /30G
- 2 tablespoons of fresh lemon juice /30ML
- 2 tablespoons extra virgin olive oil /30ML
- 3 cloves of garlic, minced

Instructions:

1) Place all ingredients inside a Ziploc bag and marinate within the fridge for 2 hours.
2) Preheat the air fryer to 390° F or 199°C .
3) Place the grill pan in the air fryer.
4) Grill the skirt steak for 20 minutes.

5) Flip the steak every 10 minutes for even grilling.

Nutrition information:

- Calories per serving: 697
- Carbs: 10.2g
- Protein:62.7 g
- Fat: 45g

Grilled Steak on Tomato-Olive Salad

Servings per Recipe: 5

Cooking Time: 50 minutes

Ingredients:

- ¼ cup extra virgin olive oil /62.5ML
- ¼ teaspoon cayenne pepper /32.5G
- ½ cup green olives, pitted and sliced /65G
- 1 cup red onion, chopped /130G
- 1 tablespoon oil /15ML
- 1 teaspoon paprika /5G
- 2 ½ pound flank /1125G
- 2 pounds cherry tomatoes, halved /900G
- 2 tablespoons Sherry vinegar /30ML
- Salt and pepper to taste

Instructions:

1) Preheat air fryer to 390° F or 199°C .
2) Place the grill pan in the air fryer.
3) Season the steak with salt, pepper, paprika, and red pepper cayenne. Brush with oil
4) Place the grill pan in the air fryer and cook for 45 to 50 minutes.
5) Meanwhile, prepare the salad by mixing the remaining ingredients.

6) Serve the beef with salad.

Nutrition information:

- Calories per serving: 351
- Carbs: 8g
- Protein: 30g
- Fat: 22g

Grilled Tri-Tip over Beet Salad

Servings per Recipe: 6

Cooking Time: 45 minutes

Ingredients:

- 1 bunch arugula, torn
- 1 bunch scallions, chopped
- 1-pound tri-tip, sliced /450G
- 2 tablespoons essential olive oil /30ML
- 3 beets, peeled and sliced thinly
- 3 tablespoons balsamic vinegar /45ML
- Salt and pepper to taste

Instructions:

1) Preheat air fryer to 390° F or 199°C .
2) Place the grill pan in the air fryer.
3) Season the tri-tip with salt and pepper. Drizzle with oil.
4) Grill for 15 minutes per batch.
5) Meanwhile, prepare the salad by mixing the remaining ingredients in a salad bowl.
6) Place in the grilled tri-trip and sprinkle with additional balsamic vinegar.

Nutrition information:

- Calories per serving: 221

- Carbs: 20.7g
- Protein: 17.2g
- Fat: 7.7g

Ground Beef on Deep Dish Pizza

Servings per Recipe: 4

Cooking Time: 25 minutes

Ingredients:

- 1 can (10-3/4 ounces) condensed tomato soup, undiluted /322.5ML
- 1 can (8 ounces) mushroom stems and pieces, drained / 240G
- 1 cup shredded part-skim mozzarella cheese /130G
- 1 cup domestic hot water (110°F to 115°F) /250ML
- 1 package (1/4 ounce) active dry yeast /7.5G
- 1 small green pepper, julienned
- 1 teaspoon dried rosemary, crushed /5G
- 1 teaspoon each dried basil, oregano and thyme /5G
- 1 teaspoon salt /5G
- 1 teaspoon sugar /5G
- 1/4 teaspoon garlic powder /1.25G
- 1-pound ground beef, cooked and drained /450G
- 2 tablespoons canola oil /30G
- 2-1/2 cups all-purpose flour /325G

Instructions:

1) Dissolve yeast in hot water, add sugar, salt, oil and 2 cups of flour. Whisk until smooth. Add the remaining flour to form a soft dough. Cover and let it sit for 20 Minutes. Divide into two and store half inside the freezer for future use.
2) Sprinkle a flat surface with flour. Place flour on it and knead into a square. Transfer into a greased air fryer baking pan. Sprinkle with beef.
3) Mix the seasonings and soup well inside a small bowl and pour over beef.
4) Sprinkle the top with mushrooms and green pepper. Top with cheese.
5) Cover the pan with foil.
6) Cook on 390° F or 199°C for 15 minutes,
7) Remove foil, cook for another 10 minutes or until cheese is melted.
8) Serve and enjoy.

Nutrition Information:

- Calories per Serving: 362
- Carbs: 39.0g
- Protein: 20.0g
- Fat: 14.0g

Ground Beef, Rice 'n Cabbage Casserole

Servings per Recipe: 6

Cooking Time: 50 minutes

Ingredients:

- 1-pound ground beef /450G
- 1 (14 ounces) can beef broth /420ML
- 1/2 cup chopped onion /65G
- 1/2 (29 ounces) can tomato sauce /870ML
- 1/2 cup uncooked white rice /65G
- 1/2 teaspoon salt /2.5G
- 1-3/4 pounds chopped cabbage /787.5G

Instructions:

1) Grease baking pan of air fryer lightly with cooking spray. Add beef and cook for 10 minutes at 360° F. stir and crumble the beef halfway through cooking time.
2) Whisk salt, rice, cabbage, onion, and tomato sauce in a bowl. Add meat and mix well. Pour in the broth.
3) Cover the pan with foil.
4) Cook for 25 minutes at 330° F or 166°C , uncover, mix and cook for another 15 minutes.
5) Serve and enjoy

Nutrition Information:

- Calories per Serving: 356
- Carbs: 25.5g
- Protein: 17.1g
- Fat: 20.6g

Sausage 'n Rice Bake from Mexico

Servings per Recipe: 4

Cooking Time: 45 minutes

Ingredients:

1/2-pound ground pork breakfast sausage /225G

1/2 (16 ounces) jar Picante sauce /480ML

1/2 (large) container sour cream

1-1/3 cups water /333ML

1/4-pound Cheddar cheese, shredded /112.5G

2/3 cup uncooked long-grain white rice /88G

Instructions:

1) Put water in a saucepan, bring to boil, stir in the rice. Cover and simmer for 20 minutes until all liquid is absorbed. Turn off fire and fluff rice.

2) Using a cooking spray, grease the baking pan of the air fryer lightly. Stir in cooked rice, sour cream, and Picante sauce. Mix well. Top with a sprinkle of cheese. Cook for 15 at 390° F or 199°C until tops are lightly browned.

3) Serve and enjoy

Nutrition Information:

- Calories per Serving: 452
- Carbs: 31.0g
- Protein: 18.9g
- Fat: 28.0g

Scallion Sauce on Lemongrass-Chili Marinated Tri-Tip

Servings per Recipe: 4

Cooking Time: 20 Minutes

Ingredients:

- 1 cup canned unsweetened coconut milk /250ML
- 2 tablespoons packed light brown sugar /30G
- 1 tablespoon fresh lime juice /15ML
- 6 garlic cloves
- 4 red or green Thai chiles, stemmed
- 2 lemongrass stalks, bottom third only, tough outer layers removed
- 1-pound tri-tip fat cap left on, cut into 1-inch cubes /450G
- 1 1 1/2" piece ginger, peeled
- 1/4 cup fish sauce /62.5ML

Scallion Dip Ingredients:

- 15 scallions, very thinly sliced
- 3 tablespoons grapeseed oil /45ML
- 2 tablespoons black vinegar /30ML
- 2 tablespoons toasted sesame seeds /30ML
- 1/4 cup fish sauce /62.5ML

Basting Sauce Ingredients:

- 1 1/2 tablespoons fresh lime juice /22.5ML
- 1/2 cup canned unsweetened coconut milk/125ML
- 2 garlic cloves, crushed
- 3 tablespoons fish sauce /45ML

Instructions:

1) Add all ingredients apart from the meat into a blender. Blend until smooth. Transfer in a bowl, place in the fridge and allow to marinate overnight.
2) 2)Mix all scallion dip Ingredients well and set aside.
3) In a separate bowl mix all basting sauce Ingredients.
4) Thread meat into skewers and set on skewer rack in the air fryer. Baste with sauce.
5) Cook for 10 minutes at 390° F or 199°C or to preferred doneness. After 5 minutes of cooking baste again and turnover skewers.
6) Using the dip as a side, serve and enjoy.

Nutrition Information:

- Calories per Serving: 579
- Carbs: 15.3g
- Protein: 32.0g
- Fat: 43.3g

Seasoned Ham 'n Mushroom Egg Bake

Servings per Recipe: 2

Cooking Time: 8 minutes

Ingredients:

- 2 eggs
- Pinch of salt
- ½ cup ham, diced /130G
- 2 mushrooms, sliced
- 1 stalk green onions, chopped
- 1 teaspoon McCormick Good Morning Breakfast Seasoning - Garden Herb /5G
- 1/4 cup milk /62.5G
- 1/4 cup shredded cheese /32.5G

Instructions:

1) Using a cooking spray, oil the baking pan lightly. Spread ham on it, then mushrooms and cheese.
2) Whisk eggs well. Season with salt and McCormick. Add milk and whisk well again. Pour over mixture in air fryer pan.
3) For 8 minutes, cook at 330° F or 166°C .
4) Sprinkle green onions and let it sit for a minute or two
5) Serve and enjoy

Nutrition Information:

- Calories per Serving: 209
- Carbs: 3.5g
- Protein: 21.5g
- Fat: 12.1g

Shepherd's Pie Made of Ground Lamb

Servings per Recipe: 4

Cooking Time: 50 minutes

Ingredients:

- 1-pound lean ground lamb /450G
- 2 tablespoons and a pair of teaspoons all-purpose flour /30G
- salt and ground black pepper to taste
- 1 teaspoon minced fresh rosemary /5G
- 2 tablespoons cream cheese /30G
- 2 ounces Irish cheese (including Dubliner®), shredded /60G
- salt and ground black pepper to taste
- 1 tablespoon milk /15ML
- 1-1/2 teaspoons olive oil /7.5ML
- 1-1/2 teaspoons butter /7.5G
- 1/2 onion, diced
- 1/2 teaspoon paprika /2.5G
- 1-1/2 teaspoons ketchup /7.5ML
- 1-1/2 cloves garlic, minced
- 1/2 (12 ounces) package frozen peas and carrots, thawed /360G
- 1-1/2 teaspoons butter /7.5G
- 1/2 pinch ground red pepper cayenne

- 1/2 egg yolk
- 1-1/4 cups water, or when needed /212.5
- 1-1/4 pounds Yukon Gold potatoes, peeled and halved /562.5G
- 1/8 teaspoon ground cinnamon /0.625G

Instructions:

1) Add water to a saucepan, add salt, bring to a boil and add potatoes. Simmer for 15 minutes until tender.
2) Meanwhile, lightly grease the baking pan of the air fryer with butter. Melt for 2 minutes at 360° F or 183°C .
3) Add ground lamb and onion. Cook for 10 minutes, stirring and crumbling halfway through cooking time.
4) Add garlic, ketchup, cinnamon, paprika, rosemary, black pepper, salt, and flour. Mix well and cook for 3 minutes.
5) Add water and deglaze pan. Continue cooking for 6 minutes.
6) Stir in carrots and peas. Evenly spread mixture in pan.
7) Once potatoes are cooked, drain well and transfer to a bowl. Mash potatoes and stir in Irish cheese, cream cheese, cayenne, and butter. Mix well. Season with pepper and salt to taste.
8) Whisk milk and egg yolk. Stir into mashed potatoes.
9) Top the ground lamb mixture with mashed potatoes.
10) Cook for 15minutes or until the top of the potatoes are lightly browned.

11) Serve, eat and enjoy

Nutrition Information:

- Calories per Serving: 485
- Carbs: 28.3g
- Protein: 29.2g
- Fat: 28.3g

Sherry 'n Soy Garlicky Steak

Servings per Recipe: 3

Cooking Time: 50 minutes

Ingredients:

- 1 tablespoon brown sugar /15G
- ½ teaspoon dry mustard /2.5G
- 1 clove of garlic, minced /
- 1 ½ pounds beef top round steak /675G
- 2 green onions, chopped
- 1/3 cup soy sauce /88ML
- 1/3 cup dry sherry /43G

Instructions:

1) Place all ingredients apart from the green onions in the Ziploc bag and allow to marinate inside the fridge for some hours.
2) Preheat the air fryer to 390° F or 199°C .
3) Place the grill pan accessory in the air fryer. Add meat and cover top with foil.
4) Grill for 50 minutes.
5) Flip meat for even doneness
6) Meanwhile, pour the marinade right into a saucepan and simmer for 10 until the sauce thickens.
7) Baste the meat with all the sauce and garnish it with green onions before serving.

Nutrition information:

- Calories per serving: 170
- Carbs: 3g
- Protein: 28g
- Fat: 5g

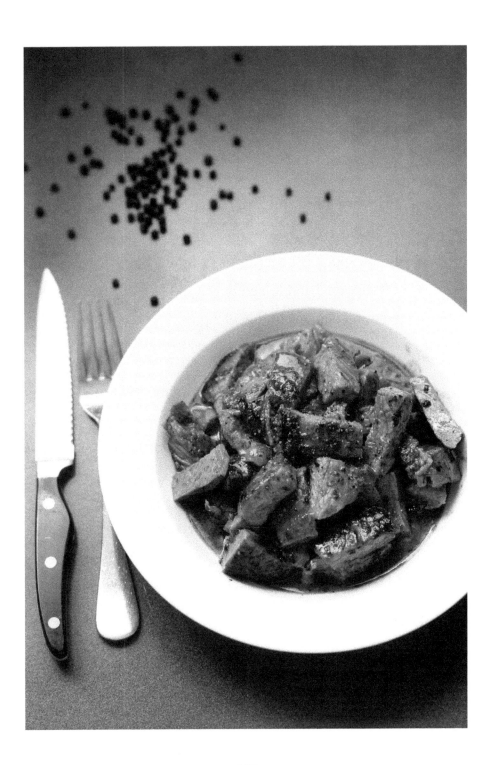

Simple Garlic 'n Herb Meatballs

Servings per Recipe: 4

Cooking Time: 20 minutes

Ingredients:

- 1 clove of garlic, minced
- 1 egg, beaten
- 1 tablespoon breadcrumbs or flour /15G
- 1 teaspoon dried mixed herbs /5G
- 1-pound lean ground beef /450G

Instructions:

1) Place all ingredients in the mixing bowl and mix using your hands.
2) Roll the mixture in your hands to form a ball, put them in the fridge to set.
3) Preheat the air fryer to 390° F or 199°C .
4) Place the meatballs in an air fryer basket and cook for 20 Minutes.
5) Shake the air fryer basket to achieve even doneness.

Nutrition information:

- Calories per serving: 599
- Carbs: 16.7g
- Protein: 54.9g
- Fat: 34.7g

Lightning Source UK Ltd.
Milton Keynes UK
UKHW020626140621
385475UK00001B/150